TABLE OF CONTENT

Before I begin, explaining to you all the importance of habits in our daily lives, I wanted to take a minute to share my gratitude with Mary Morley, the kind soul who encouraged me to publish this book. I am not a writer by trade. I work with people, people like you, maybe. The people I work with struggle with change and lack the guidance necessary for their ultimate success. I offer that guidance.

I never sought to write a book at all. This book is a collection of techniques I use in my work. It was Mary who encouraged me to put it in the form you will see here. She thought that maybe it was possible to take these techniques I had developed and publish them in a way that would be helpful to those who don't understand just how large an impact habits have in our daily lives.

It is with that spirit that I published Habits for Weight Loss and & Healthy Living. I hope you will forgive me should I struggle at times to communicate as effectively as you would like. If you have questions, I urge you to contact me at the Facebook page Morley Publishing set up for this project.

I am confident I can help you comprehend the importance of habits and how to master them to change your life. I have done it countless times in the real world and I am sure I can have the same success through this book.

Introduction

I hope if you are reading this book it's because you are looking to make permanent healthy changes in your life. I can imagine this isn't the first time you have tried to make these changes. After all, I know from personal experience, the trials of struggling with creating healthy and positive habits when I'd rather just sit lazily on the couch, eat my pizza and drink my soda. I spent years, in fact, teaching others about changing habits in their lives before I was successful in changing the negative habits in my own. You don't truly understand the height of hypocrisy until you weigh 350 pounds and are lecturing a person with developmental disabilities about healthy choices and portion control. We all know, on some level, what is required to lose weight and what defines a healthy life, but it's what isn't black and white, what isn't written in bold letters right in front of our faces, that keeps us from being successful.

This is not a diet book. You won't learn about low calorie foods or menu plans. I won't compare the south beach and Atkins diets'. Any sensible diet can be used to successfully lose weight. This is not a book discussing the pros and the cons of exercise. Any exercise is beneficial and can serve your purpose.

The reason we won't focus on these ideas in this book is because we want to address the overall issues preventing us from making permanent positive changes in our life. Until we learn to make these permanent changes, no diet or exercise program will work long term. Sure, you may lose some weight for a while, but as is usually the case, a few months down the road you will gain it all back.

I want you to know that I understand fully the struggle you are facing. I have lived your struggle. I am, at times, still living the struggle. I know what it feels like to fail time and time again. I know the negative reinforcement we receive daily from all directions. It feels at times almost like an assault. We are inundated with unhealthy choices and it takes all of our willpower to resist them. It can be that pizza commercial on our way home from work or the peer pressure to go out drinking all night instead of going to the gym. In my experience, if there is a temptation to give into, I will find a way. I have in the past, and this continues to be a struggle. We struggle with being healthy only to, at some point in time, fall to these temptations due to momentary weaknesses. Each time we fail, it feels like it is that much harder to begin again. I have lost the weight. I have gained it back. I have lost it again. At one point in my life, I weighed over 350 pounds. Through shear willpower, as many of you have, I lost a great deal of it, over 80 pounds in fact, only to gain it all back and then some after my father died. We are human and we can't use only willpower to make healthy choices, because at some point, we will be weak and fail. No, we need the knowledge of why, at our moments of weakness, we fail. We need to learn about habits, how they are formed and how they affect everything we do. It is in this understanding that we gain the superhuman power of making healthy choices consistently, in spite of the real life distractions and barriers we face. Does that sound too good to be true? It isn't. We will learn how to change these negatives into positives. First, I want to go into my personal background, and hopefully give you an understanding of why I do what I do and why I believe I can help you.

I have worked in human services for over a decade. I have worked individually with hundreds of people, from all backgrounds, in all situations. We have spent thousands of hours together, going over choices. I have written hundreds of plans and been involved in several hundred more planning meetings. In these meetings, everyone's discussing what this particular person should do to achieve this outcome or that skill. These meetings would be fantastic, if they were what determined success or failure, but they aren't. We all have these meetings within ourselves, in our own minds all of the time. We will say, I need to lose weight, or I really need to start exercising more. Smokers constantly say they should quit smoking. A hung-over college student says he will never drink again. I don't know how many times I quit drinking in college, but I know I quit a lot! There is a disconnect between when these meetings occur, whether they involve behavior specialists and residential coordinators, or an internal discussion with yourself; and the execution of these grand plans. We know what we are supposed to do. If we want to lose weight, we know we need to eat less or exercise more. So why don't we?

Knowing the action we should take for a positive outcome is miles away from consistently making the correct choice to affect positive changes in our lives. It took me many years, a great many "failures" and some fantastic mentors before I finally understood just how deeply ingrained our behaviors are, and how we need to approach changing them.

The reason we are overweight and living an unhealthy lifestyle is that we have been conditioned to make poor choices practically our entire life. Our decisions are based almost entirely on habits that we have developed. Once I realized how entrenched these habits are in us, and that they are the reason we fail over and over again, I could finally grasp how to make real change in lives, both in the lives of people I was working with, and in my own.

With this knowledge in hand, we started developing plans that would address negative habits in people. We would strive for awareness and consistency in everything that we were doing. By creating plans tailored to the negative habits of each individual and identifying the triggers, we were able to create real change in many of the people we were working with.

Almost anyone reading this book, who is overweight, or struggling with making healthy lifestyle changes, can tell you they eat too much, or don't exercise enough. They can tell you they drink too much or that they shouldn't eat out as often as they do. There are many things that we realize we should or shouldn't do, but very few people can identify the habits and situations that cause us to make these poor decisions on a daily basis. The reason is that 90% of what we do is performed by habit. Habits are a form of "cruise control" for the brain. If you have ever done well on a diet for a week and had something unexpected come up that caused you to fail on your diet, this was a negative habit that unexpectedly wrecked all of your hard work because you weren't prepared for it, and your mind took advantage of your moment of weakness.

Maybe you have tried several different diets, such as Atkins or the South Beach diet. Maybe you bought your gym memberships every year, and just failed to use it as often as necessary. The reasons why these diets succeed or fail or an exercise plan is successful or not, is based entirely on how effective the plans are on establishing new positive habits in our lives. The problem is this only addresses the issue of positive habits; it doesn't address our negative habits that will continue to derail us.

Perhaps you are reading this as part of a New Year's resolution, or as you prepare for a vacation to the beach, with your family. This time it can be different. Devote yourself to understanding the habits that hold you back, addressing them, as well as establishing new positive habits. In doing so, we will be successful, together.

In this book we will learn together how to identify our habits. We will work on adapting our habits to improve our quality of life and make these habits work for us instead of against us.

The truth is losing weight is the same as accomplishing anything. We have to put in the work to accomplish the goal. The problem is a lot of us don't know what that work is. Don't worry though; it's been my experience, that it's a lot easier once you understand what is required. Real permanent changes are possible, with the right guidance. I promise we will get there.

As we progress in this book, we will cover all that I have discovered over the last 15 years of investigating the science behind the habits of healthy living. We will begin by understanding why we are overweight. We will cover habits at great length. How the body develops habits. We will move on to identifying our habits. Then, we will learn steps to take to understand how these habits affect us, on a personal level. We will analyze some of the most common negative habits and how we can change them to make permanent positive life changes, changes that will stay with us forever.

We will discuss establishing positive changes in our lives. You will learn how to develop new positive habits, easily and quickly, with very little effort. Once you understand the steps to creating a habit, and how to remain consistent in your endeavor, you will see how positive an impact creating these habits will have on your life.

We will discover "food addiction." We will discuss the reasons why certain foods have a hold on us, and how we can break that chain of control. We will go in depth about the way the body processes food and the reasons for those insatiable cravings that many of us feel. We will learn how to identify these cravings as they are happening, and we will learn techniques to cut these cravings off before they derail our progress.

Finally in Habits for Weight Loss & Healthy Living, we will identify the entire process to change. We will learn to track and change our negative habits and we will learn about some of the pitfalls in the struggle for permanent healthy change. We will discuss the hardest parts of this journey, and how you handle setbacks to ensure success in your efforts.

If you are reading this book, it is most likely because you are overweight or unhealthy and want to change. I also know that most people struggle with these changes. Once you understand how the mind controls the body and everything we do, success is within reach! I promise you, read this book. Learn about the habits of healthy living. Finally, take the steps that I outline in this book to make the necessary changes in your life. Nothing could be more important. Following these steps will do so much more than just allow you to finally lose your excess weight! Learning how to control your habits will change all aspects of your life. I learned these processes through education and trial and error. Nothing is ever easy, but this is a process to success, I truly believe will affect the same positive change in you, as it has in me, and the people I work with every day.

We are going to take this journey together. We will address why we struggle and how we will overcome each problem as it arises, together. I want to be clear about what this book is. It is a guide; it will show you the steps to permanent and positive change. This book will provide a very good basis for changing your life. However, it can't possibly answer every question or solve every situation. In these cases, when you are really struggling, or just need some positive reinforcement, I urge you to join us on Facebook. Come join our small but growing and dedicated community, as we explore the need for change, and the best practices for changing these negative habits. I am active on the page. I promise I will help, if at all possible, in clarifying any questions you may have or even just discuss the trials of change. We've all been there, and we can succeed if we are willing to be positive and consistent. The greatest part of this journey is that you aren't going alone, and people have gone before you. The path lies before us. Let's get started.

Why People Struggle Making Changes

We like to think that we, as humans, are independent thinkers, and that our consciousness is used to make every decision. We believe we are capable of anything at any time, but most of us fail to understand just how much we rely on our subconscious to carry out the daily activities of our lives. As you will come to understand, these habits control almost every part of what we do. In fact, our mind relies very heavily on these habits, so it can focus on immediate and pressing dangers, or on things that require a great deal of concentration. Because of the need for relying on these habits, we have evolved to live very repetitious lifestyles. We eat at the same times, work at the same times, sleep at the same times and perform other activities, all as part of a routine. Of course, there are exceptions, but you will find that a great deal of what you do on a daily basis is the same, almost every day.

So what happens, when there are changes to our routine? Unfortunately, we don't handle unknowns very well. When we are faced with these changes, the body undergoes stress. The levels of stress vary, depending on our comfort levels, but it is nevertheless, an uncomfortable experience. Now, the mind struggles to gain as much pleasure and to limit as much pain as possible, this is known as the pleasure principle.

Because of this principle, we find it hard to make the positive changes we want, due to our mind fighting against us to prevent the stress that occurs during changes. In fact, this stress is the same, if to a lesser extent, as the withdrawal stress felt by people trying to quit smoking or drinking. What is an addiction, but an incredibly strong habit, which gives a larger reward when we participate? So, you understand, we are fighting ourselves.

So how exactly does this affect our losing weight? This is a clouded issue, made so mainly to confuse people into wasting their money buying useless products. The truth is, that while there are some products that are designed to legitimately help us along in the process of losing weight, many more are designed to be a flashy product, selling us on the fallacy that losing weight is about anything other than learning how to establish good healthy habits. The industry of weight loss thrives on misinformation and confusion. If these companies can keep us in the dark, thinking that we can go on doing what we've been doing, but just take this pill every day, we will lose weight and get healthy; they will continue to sell more pills. They are selling the dream of health, which would be fine if they provided an actual solution, but in most cases, they fail us.

So how did we become overweight to begin with? It's really quite simple. How did we develop these negative habits? We are overweight because we eat too much; any person who is overweight knows this. Each person burns a certain amount of calories every day. We burn calories just surviving, that is; breathing, pumping blood, and regulating a thousand different processes in the human body. Add to that, the amount of calories we burn being physically active. Walking, running, lifting, anything that we physically do, burns additional calories. If we eat more calories than we burn on a daily basis, we will gain weight. Conversely, if we want to lose weight, we simply need to eat fewer calories. This is pretty common knowledge, but why now, as opposed to other times in history, is our society facing this obesity epidemic?

The number of calories that we as humans burn has declined steadily since we moved from hunter gatherers to farmers, and has declined even more since the evolution of the free market system. It is more productive to be good at less, and trade for what was needed, instead of being responsible for all of our own living requirements. We have evolved to make life easier for ourselves, and in the process, we have contributed to the cause of this obesity epidemic.

This is just one part of the double edged sword! With the simplification of life, that is, making survival easier, food has been provided for us in great abundance. Our mind is struggling to catch up. Throughout our evolution, we ate when we had food available, and stored the excess so that when we reached periods of little food, we could survive. We no longer face these long periods of famine, at least in developed countries. Everywhere we go, we are being offered way more than we need for such small amounts of money. We feel genetically obligated to eat in excess.

To this evolutionary hurdle, we add the need for businesses to increase their profits and sales. In an effort to increase their business, these companies are relying on questionable, possible underhanded, techniques. Restaurants and food manufacturers are using psychology and chemistry to manipulate us into buying more food and more often. This manipulation has invaded every aspect of our culture. It is now quite common for people to eat out every single day, or rarely eat a normal, meals worth of calories. These changes, without even realizing it, have placed us on the path to obesity. Without educating ourselves, and making much needed changes in the way we approach food, we will continue heading down this path.

All of these negative habits we have developed have to be addressed, one at a time, with conscious dedication, by each of us. Remember however, this isn't an easy process. We have to fight our ingrained routines. Our subconscious doesn't give up easily. We must focus on changing our habits, one at a time. It will be a struggle, but I can show you how to create the positive new habits we need, and how to address our negative habits that are holding us back.

Habits

Now, to be successful in our endeavor to lose weight, we have to understand the power of habits. Habits control 90% of everything we do. What started out as a process the brain used to save energy, has become an autopilot for our lives; meaning that we actually have very little control over what we do each moment, and we are often unaware. When and how we go to the bathroom, when and how we eat, how we drive, the first few minutes at work, even how we workout and relax can all be practically mindless (subconscious) activities for us.

It is important to understand that habits control who we are, what we accomplish and how we behave when facing any situation. We are overweight because a series of habits we hold, lead us to make choices where we eat more calories than we burn. It can be one major habit such as drinking too much soda at certain times each day or it can be small habits such as eating a cookie when we get to work in the morning and going out to eat on days when you work late. What if we controlled these habits? What if instead of eating that extra cookie or drinking that soda, we established drinking 12 ounces of water to replace the soda or the cookie. That single change in habit can help us lose a significant amount of weight. The fact is habits determine if we are making positive or negative strides. We are the sum of the habits we have developed. If we choose to reinforce positive habits, we will make positive strides. That is the goal of this book.

Have you ever wondered why weight loss programs like Atkins or the South Beach diet work for some people and not others? How about workout programs like P90x? These programs only work as well as they can establish positive habits for the people using the program. The Atkins diet specifies time frames and steps, over the course of a long period of time because it is this set system that reinforces establishing positive habits. Why does P90x last for 90 days? Despite their muscle confusion plan, working out on a set schedule for 90 days works, because after 90 days of being consistent, it is habitual that you will work out hard every day, allowing you to keep these healthy changes permanently. Make no mistake however, once you stop cutting out all those carbs, or stop the P90x routine without replacing the workout, you will undo all of your successes. We are going right to the source in this book. Rather than offer you a plan that just hopes to establish positive habits, you will learn how to change negative habits as well. With the information in this book, you can be successful with any diet or exercise program, a professional one such as the ones listed above or one you set for yourself. As long as you understand the most important thing in weight loss is consistency, and establishing positive habits while eliminating negative habits, you can control the conditions in which you succeed.

What Makes Up a Habit?

Habits are a way for the subconscious to conserve energy while performing daily tasks. The body "programs" itself to perform certain steps based on situations that occur, very much like a computer program. The three steps to a habit are called the habit loop.

The cue, or the catalyst, is what occurs that sets in motion the habit. Let's say you see a cookie. The mind recognizes this situation and put's into motion the routine.

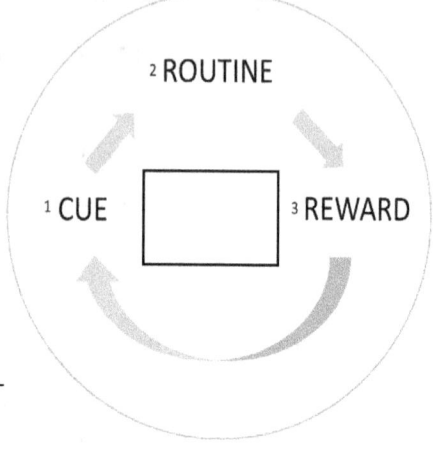

The routine is the action of the habit. You see the cookie and then you eat the cookie. Your body recognizes that you successfully completed a task, so you go get a snack to take a short break.

The reward in these scenarios is the feel good chemicals released by the cookie to the brain, or a quick energy spike.

Every habit consists of these 3 parts, the cue, the routine and the reward. What we need to do to successfully lose weight is, to address the routine. To do that however, we need to understand the whole process. We need to know what our cue factors are for eating that cookie. The hardest part is defining these terms in each individual case because everyone is different. We will discuss how to identify cues and routines and how to address them to transform negative habits into positive ones.

How powerful are habits? They are responsible for everything that we do! Think about that. The truth is we can change almost anything about ourselves simply by changing negative habits or establishing new and positive ones. Once you unlock the knowledge to address your habits, you can do much more than just lose weight. You can become a more effective student, a better worker. Ever struggle with motivation? Do you think of yourself as a procrastinator? These are just bad habits mislabeled by convenient words.

So let's take some time to identify different habits. For example, maybe after you get home from work you grab some chips and sit down to watch television. You can decide for yourself whether this is a good habit for yourself or not, but I dare say it may be something we can address. After you sit down, eat and watch television you don't have motivation to do the laundry. There are a couple habits taking place here. The grabbing food is a habit; sitting down to watch TV is a habit, both triggered by returning home from work. The habit when returning home from work is shutting down, going in to sleep mode. It isn't a lack of motivation as much as, you've trained your body to shut down after work. If, when you return home from work, you immediately start your laundry instead of grabbing your chips, you will begin to establish the new habit of being productive after returning home, instead of shutting down. It will take time, it will most likely be uncomfortable, as changing any habit usually is, but with consistency, it will no longer be uncomfortable. In fact, you will consider the new habit of being productive after work, as being second nature, much the way the old habit was.

What Do Habits Control?

Habits make up the majority of everything we do. From when we sleep, to what we eat. How we respond to meeting people is habit, or how we study for a test. Some people like watching TV in the dark, others like going to the grocery store at night. These are all habits. Think of the morning routine. Personally, I wake up, generally between 7 and 7:30, use the bathroom, stumble downstairs, start the coffee and take my black lab outside. We come back in, and I feed my black lab and my kitty hellion. I sit down, take a drink of coffee and have my first real thought of the day, about what work needs to be done. All of the above is habitual behavior.

Habits are everywhere in our daily life. We have a habit for everything. We have habits for when we wake up, habits for what we do when we first enter our car or on our way to work. Generally speaking, the first 15 minutes at work each day, are habitually the same every single day.

Habits are programmed responses. They aren't limited to what we do when we arrive at work or when we wake up. They are present when we succeed, when we fail, when we are stressed or when we are tired. Habits take over when we anticipate trying something new, or when we are faced with something that we don't like. In all of these areas, habits are such a strong force that if we stop to consider this fact for a minute, it scares us. We as humans are so comfortable being creatures of free will! We have boundless intelligence and knowledge; we could leave our house today and drive 6 hours to the mountains, or the beach, or the desert. We could call in and quit our job or we just up and change careers at a whim. We could do so very much, in fact we often say we are going to, right? Then, why is it that we don't? It is simply because of our habits. We are habitual creatures, in everything that we do, and ignoring these routines is extremely difficult. Unfortunately, until we address them, we won't obtain the success that we really want, whether it is in our career, in relationships or in weight loss. So how do we develop habits?

How Are Habits Developed?

Habits are a cycle of learned behavior. To repeat again, each habit consists of a cue, a routine and a reward. Habits are developed because when something occurs, we respond by responding with some action. This creates a pleasurable sensation in the brain, often by the release of chemicals such as serotonin, or the prevention of stress causing chemicals such as cortisol.

Habits are formed simply by repeated behavior in such situations. For example, let's set out to establish the habit of exercise right when we wake up in the morning. We have the cue we want to establish an action upon, notably when we wake up. What routine do we want to establish? We want to exercise. It doesn't matter what exercise it is. It can be sit ups and pushups, a walk or run around the block or walking up and down stairs. The reward is the easy part. The body takes care of it for us. Exercise increases endorphins and serotonin, feel good and stress relieving chemicals, in the brain. Now, repeat. Repetition is necessary. However, it is easier to begin new positive habits than it is to transform old negative habits.

Eventually, this becomes habit. There have been many studies on establishing habits. Some have hypothesized it takes 21 days to create a habit, others that 27 days are linked to muscle memory. The truth is you won't even notice it has become a habit until someone mentions it down the road. When I first started tracking my calories daily, I set out with the goal to track every calorie for 21 days in a row. I didn't realize I had been successful until I was helping a client on day 45 and she asked me how I made sure I didn't eat too much. It felt so amazing to successfully set such a positive habit that I immediately set out to affect more positive habits in my life.

This is an important thing to consider as you begin your journey to establishing new habits. The great thing about habits is that they build on themselves. Exercise will no longer be a struggle after you have established the habit of exercise, in fact you will feel the stress, if you have to one day, skip a workout. After successfully creating this habit, you will set out to establish other positive habits related to it, continually improving yourself, and in the process it becomes almost easy!

Before we can start establishing some of the positive habits that will help improve our lives, we need to make ourselves aware of the habits we already have. We became obese because of our negative habits, not because of our positive ones.

The problem with habits is that they are incredibly difficult to break. What we will focus on is identifying some of our bad habits and reprogramming ourselves to have a different routine reaction to the trigger (cue).

So How Do We Change these Self-Destructive Habits?

It is important to note before we move on to the next chapter, that it is almost impossible to get rid of bad habits. Many of us know that one person, who was a smoker, who quit for a decade or more only to start up again. They weren't prepared for some situation that arose and that led them to start smoking again. Once they gave in again, without the information and resolve necessary, that is provided by the information in this book, they were unable to keep from falling back into the trap, which is smoking addiction. Habits are part of who we are and unless we are properly prepared for their power over us, we will succumb to them. Part of that preparation is learning to identify each habit, the good and the bad. We do that with the knowledge that everything we do is habit, and take the time to identify each of the parts. I list some of the most common negative habits that relate to losing weight and making healthy choices in a future chapter. However each person must take time to realize how habits are affecting themselves. Once we have identified our bad habits, we can go about addressing them.

It is impossible to get rid of a bad habit. Once the habit is ingrained in our mind, it is there forever. These habits are learned. Because they are learned, we are capable of retraining them with directed effort. No matter how strong our subconscious is, our concerted effort and mindfulness is strong enough to change these habits. By identifying our habits and all their parts and determining the best way to manipulate them, we can make positive changes in our daily routines. We make our mind work for us in weight loss and healthy living.

Reprogramming Bad Habits

Once we have identified our bad habits and have labeled them, we have an understanding of what triggers our worst habits. For example, after a stressful day, our mind tells us to eat a double helping of ice cream, because it releases chemicals in the brain, giving the body the same feeling as a drug addict taking a hit of their drug of choice. Food is the drug of choice for a lot of us. So we know that we eat high calorie ice cream after having a stressful day at work to receive our heavy dose of feel good chemicals. That is a fully identified habit. Now we set about re-programming this habit.

It is important to remember that reprogramming a habit takes time. It has been written about and hypothesized over and over again about how long it takes. Some say 21 days, others a month. I maintain that it varies based entirely on how ingrained the habit is and how dedicated and successful we are at the reprogram-ming process. I like to say that you should start out with a goal. Let's aim for 21 days, once we hit 21 days we give ourselves a pat on the back! Good Job Us! Then we aim for 30 days. Again, we celebrate the victory at 30 days, but we continue. See, the truth is that to be successful, to successfully reprogram our bad habit is to forget that we are trying to reprogram the habit. Remember, we don't consciously perform our habits, they are part of us.

I like to refer to my first success at reprogramming habits. I was aiming to track how many calories I ate a day, every day. I would weigh my food, log it on a website and compare it versus my dai-ly goals. I did exactly as I stated above. My goal was 21 days. The next thing I knew, when I was helping a client with weight loss, we were discussing tracking calories when I suddenly realized I had successfully counted my calories for 45 days straight, without even realizing it. This is victory! This is where we should aim to be, no matter what habit we are trying to change or how we are replacing it.

We have to determine how to best proceed at reprogramming bad habits. To start, let's choose one bad habit. Let's pick one of the big ones. Once we go through the process of identifying habits, you will understand more clearly what you want to focus on first. These are the macro habits that affect us on several levels. We want to choose something that, when successful, we can build on that makes a greater and more positive change in our lives.

When I first started, I started with three habits' I wanted to adjust or establish. I wanted to create the habit of tracking my food intake. This was a new habit to me, but it allowed me to remain conscious of my food choices throughout the day, as well as to provide data to show me the cause and effect of the choices I made on my body.

Second, I resolved to set a schedule and a menu of what to eat each day. This was perhaps the greatest choice I could have made. Going on the AMA guide of calories for a normal weight person of my height, I designed a menu using a program caused MyFitnessPal that allowed me to track exactly how many calories I would consume on a daily basis.

I didn't utilize a specific diet. I didn't give up any foods. I simply planned and measured everything and resolved to eat on a schedule. By having a schedule, I at all times knew when I would be eating. That certainty, allowed me to break the habit of grabbing food whenever it was available, or eating whenever I felt like it.

I eliminated eating except as it pertained to my schedule, and I planned for any interruptions to my schedule that might occur.

Finally, I replaced the habit's that enabled my overeating daily. I replaced the habit of stopping at the convenience store everyday with getting to work a few minutes early. I used this time to socialize more with my coworkers, to mentally prepare for my work day, making a positive use of my time. As part of my scheduling every meal, I resolved to pack my lunch every night for the following day. While this was a struggle, as it meant giving up eating out daily with my coworkers, it allowed me to make healthy choices that I could track consistently. I scheduled a day every two weeks to go out to eat, but I planned what I was going to eat. This way, I was prepared for craving the 2000 calorie meal I would sometimes order, and could make a better decision instead.

To reprogram the negative habits into positive ones, we need to analyze daily why the changes we are making are beneficial. This is what gives us the resolve to reprogram our minds.

By tracking my daily caloric intake and keeping track of the weight I lost, I could predict goals and realistically expect to reach them. In fact, I hit every goal for the first 6 months because I could look at the numbers and have a fair expectation of my progress. I knew that every day I was losing half of a pound. I knew that as long as I tracked my calories and stuck to my calorie plan, I would continue to lose weight every day. People often times give up on a diet or plan because they don't see results as they expect to. This is in part due to unrealistic expectations, but also because they view weight loss as some magical process. It isn't. Weight loss is a scientific process that can be tracked pretty accurately. If you weigh 300 pounds and you resolve to track your calories, I can guarantee that if you eat 2000 calories a day, every day and you verify this through effective tracking, you will lose weight. A lot of people don't like this because it puts the accountability back on us. Reprogramming bad habits can only work if you are willing to dedicate yourself to it. Each day at the end of the day, I would verbally, that is out loud, compliment myself on successfully tracking my calories. Knowing that by hitting my calorie goals, I lost weight that day, I would congratulate myself on being one day closer to my goal. It is essential that you verbally praise yourself. You don't have to do it in front of other people; you can do it in bed or in the bathroom, or in your car. But do it. The process of verbally hearing that you did something well reinforces the reprogramming from the negative to the positive habit. This is mandatory. I promise you, that while you might feel silly the first time you do it, when you wake up the next morning and feel good and ready to be successful on your plan again, you will realize just how effective verbal praise is.

How to Establish Positive Habits in Our Life

So how do we establish these positive changes in our lives? We have already decided that this is what we want more than anything, but we need the resolve to keep that at the forefront of our minds, day in and day out. We need to recognize the importance of keeping this focus. The mind will dedicate its resources to what we are consistently focusing on. In fact, this is a requirement to be able to change our habits and establish new ones. Without clarity of purpose and singular focus on the changing of these habits, we will fail.

When establishing these new habits, we must make them our top priority and the most important thing in our life. That is an incredibly hard commitment. Remember, we are trying to defeat habits that have been ingrained in us for many years. The mind resists this change and it is only through constant focus that we are able to reprogram ourselves.

This is the purpose of documenting our habits and our successes and failures. Whether we succeed in our goal every day or not, this documentation keeps the transformation process at the forefront of our cognitive focus. There are other things we can do to keep this focus. An easy solution to remaining focused when creating new habits is by triggers throughout the day. For example, once we are done with our drive home from work each day, we can go for a 2 mile walk. This trigger makes it easier to program the mind with the new habit. Or we can use our cell phones, set a daily alarm and use that alarm as a trigger to establish the new desired habit. Whatever it takes, we must be mindful in the moment, as we focus on forming our new habits.

Another barrier to successfully developing new habits or defeating old habits, are distractions. We face distractions every day. Things come up at work; the people in our lives require our assistance for this thing or for that. These distractions limit our ability to remain focused on the reprogramming process. Unfortunately, we are unable to completely eliminate these distractions. Life happens, and part of this process of reprogramming is learning to deal with life on our new terms.

We have to learn to prepare for issues before they arise, as we fight our old bad habits and establish new ones. This process is fairly simple, however. Take a few minutes right now and write down some potential interruptions to your schedule. Perhaps you have to work late one day. Perhaps family activities are happening after work, and you won't have time to cook. An old friend shows up at your door. You wake up late in the morning, and won't have time for breakfast. Predict these potential barriers and then decide how you will deal with them in a positive way. By doing this you won't allow your mind to take advantage of a stressful position by making a poor decision. For example, some potential solutions to the above problems may be that there is a menu online and you can pick the healthiest meal. To prevent being forced to make bad decisions when in a hurry, keep healthy snacks available to grab quickly if you are running late so you don't end up eating 500 calories worth of subpar convenience store food on the way to work because you are starving. Preparation is the key to dealing with these distractions. Take the time now so that you aren't derailed later.

The Power of Self Positive Reinforcement

Positive reinforcement is rewarding a desired behavior. When you give a dog a treat for sitting or give a child a star for a painting, you are rewarding that behavior. Positive reinforcement has been proven to work in a myriad of situations, and though there has been some dispute as to the extent of its effectiveness, it will be a positive tool, a cornerstone to our success.

Our goal is to succeed at all costs. As I stated above, we will utilize any tool possible in this goal. So how are we going to use positive reinforcement to change our negative habits? As part of our daily tracking system we are going to include self-positive reinforcement. It is important that we not seek this positive reinforcement from others. We have to learn to be responsible to ourselves and to accomplish things for our own sake. While it is nice to receive this positive reinforcement from others, relying on it leaves us requiring that validation over and over again, and when we don't receive it we tend to falter.

We will focus on proper self-positive reinforcement, but first we have to understand why positive reinforcement works, and why it works even if we perform it on ourselves. Positive reinforcement works because we as human beings seek success, and we want to receive approval. The problem arises when we don't celebrate our triumphs, and rely on other people to give us our reinforcement. When we don't receive that approval, there is no reinforcement of positive behaviors. This is a wasted opportunity to make strides toward reconditioning the positive changes that we are seeking. The solution is awarding ourselves positive reinforcement.

There are many problems that arise when we expect praise and positive reinforcement from others. For starters, many are unaware of just how strong reinforcement can be. If everyone knew how great a tool focused positive reinforcement was, we would learn it in school as a necessary skill in working in a team environment. People are unaware. What's more, they are too busy with their own problems. We as people are extremely self-centered. While we all need to focus more on helping others, and taking into consideration how others are doing, we can't afford to ignore the world we live in. Some people may wait a long time for positive reinforcement from their family, friends and coworkers; this isn't conducive to positive and consistent change. Finally, relying on others for praise leaves us open to negative consequences that may be caused, intentionally or unintentionally by others. What if we come to expect positive praise from our boss for our work? He gives this praise often, then for whatever reason, one time, fails to offer that praise. This sends a signal to our brain that we are doing something wrong, when it may be that our boss was having a bad day, or focusing on something else. This type of miscommunication makes it hard to rely on others for something that is as important as reassurance that we are making good decisions in life. It is far better for us to reassure ourselves and celebrate our successes.

Self-positive reinforcement also helps us face a cruel world. We face negativity from the moment we enter the world, every day. We face unrealistic expectations from the media, unfair expectations at work and an intense mind draining existence at times. People can be incredibly unsupportive. People will line up to hinder your progress. You will find that some of your friends won't support your decision to get healthy. Perhaps some family members will hinder your efforts by trying to break your newly established good habits. These aren't unintentional, though they may be subconscious. These are the reactions of people who identify that you are making positive changes, and that it is easier to ridicule you for your changes than to make the changes themselves. What's more, often times this is completely subconscious. If you have a friend who is constantly trying to get you to eat a brownie at snack time, even though you have repeatedly told her that you would rather eat at a later time, this is her unconsciously pouring negativity on you. It's a tough world to make these permanent changes in. That's why we must rely on ourselves to celebrate our own victories and provide our own self-positive reinforcement. It's not always other people's fault but we can't allow them to have that kind of control over us. In the end, all that really matters anyway is how we view ourselves. If we can be proud of ourselves we have won. We must first learn then, how to celebrate victories in ourselves.

Positive reinforcement serves us many benefits on our path to losing weight. In addition to keeping our mind positively focused on the long term goal of establishing healthy habits, it lets us know when we are being successful in taking one small step at a time. Successfully completing a goal can be hard to visualize, it is important that we celebrate the small steps that add up to ultimate victory.

In addition to keeping us focused on celebrating our successes, self-positive reinforcement keeps our attention evaluating ourselves. We determine how to define success and what we need to work on to achieve that success. Unfortunately, everywhere we go, we are inundated with negativity. Whether it is in the grocery store, at the gym, at work, or in school, we will face negativity in some forms. As mentioned before, we may face it from people who are incapable of making the changes for themselves. People are threatened by others who are making positive changes in their lives, especially when they are in a stagnant place themselves. We will discuss the important of surrounding ourselves with positive and successful people. The reason why we need to surround ourselves with these people is because they, like you, will be focusing on establishing good habits to assist in their journey to becoming the best possible person they can be. Take note of this. Seek to identify these habits in people in your everyday life. As you redefine your daily habits, look to see the people who support you. You will find that they are usually working to better themselves. But when you find a lack of support, from a coworker, a friend or even a family member, you will find someone who is stuck in their routine, who isn't making the changes necessary to improve their own lives.

We focus on positive self-reinforcement so we can prevent other people from overshadowing our positives with their negatives. If we are accountable only to ourselves, no one else can be responsible for our success or failure. As this is always the case, it is important to create the habit of self-approval.

Once we understand just how important a tool self-positive reinforcement is, we have to examine how we can apply it in our lives to have a positive impact. When we talk about positive reinforcement, what exactly are we talking about? We are talking about holding ourselves accountable for every action and celebrating every positive action we make. In the scope of this book, every time we make a positive step towards establishing a positive habit, we celebrate it. This action reinforces the positive habit, and while it is not wholly responsible for the successful assimilation of the new habit into our life, it is a tool that helps a great deal. So when do we provide this action for ourselves?

The general consensus is that positive reinforcement must take place immediately after a behavior for it to have the greatest impact. However, I feel that this isn't conducive to people actually participating in the necessary activity of positive self-reinforcement. We simply aren't going to stop in the lunchroom after making a healthy choice and say out loud, "good job!" to ourselves. In my experience, the best way to approach giving ourselves this reinforcement is to, at the end of the day, say out loud, good job for every success we had for the day. Start from the beginning of your day, and review everything with an honest eye. Every time you did something positive to reinforce a positive habit, say good job and be specific. Perhaps you craved a cupcake but instead drank a glass of water, tell yourself good job for that and tell yourself why. Tell yourself that you didn't need to eat an additional 300 calories, because you had already had breakfast, and water is important for the mind and body to work well. Then move on to the next success. Even if you fell completely off the wagon, ate an entire cheese pizza after a stressful day, then skipped the gym. The mere fact that you are analyzing your day with an honest and non-judgmental way is a success. This analyzing at the end of every day is a key tool to remaining committed and consistent. Celebrate that decision.

When analyzing and giving that positive self-reinforcement, take a minute to correct any negative behaviors as well. Do it in an honest and fair way. Don't judge yourself harshly, don't scold yourself. Habits are not transformed in a day, or a week, or even a month. They are formed through constantly working positive changes. You won't succeed by punishing yourself; you can be your own best ally or your own worst enemy.

If you fail at one of the habits you are working to change or nurture, identify when you failed. For example one of habits you are nurturing is exercising every day after work. You have been doing great at it! Then one day your boss called you out for missing a deadline, in front of all of your coworkers, you had a flat tire in the morning, and you didn't sleep well the night before. So you say, forget it, go home and watch television after work. Identify the cause or causes of missing your workout and remind yourself that you physically could have worked out, everything else was an excuse not to, let's try again tomorrow. Perhaps there are other things to take away from this process. Maybe you went home to grab your workout clothes but decided you didn't feel like going back out. Well, we can address this by being sure we have our workout clothes with us in the morning so we can go right to the gym after work. Maybe we can work out with a co-worker or friend to help keep us accountable. The point of this self-analysis every night is that every success deserves a celebration, and every setback has a solution to keep it from happening again. Take the time and you will be successful over the long run.

We mentioned earlier the importance of surrounding ourselves with positive people. We discussed the difference between people striving to better themselves and others who don't, and their attitudes towards your goals. We must surround ourselves with positive people, if only as another tool to success. As I mentioned, any tool we can use to help ensure we succeed is something we must utilize. This is a war, to change our negative habits to become the person we have always wanted to be.

We must demand positivity from the people around us. We

cannot afford to have negativity seeping into our ear as we try to succeed. Negativity is a distraction to everything that we are trying to accomplish. We become what we think about. I challenge you to ignore constant negativity while trying to make positive changes. It is nearly impossible in the best of circumstances. It is a downright recipe for failure in most cases. Now, I am not saying to end your relationship with your sister because she is constantly trying to derail your diet, or to break up with your boyfriend because he tells you that exercising is a waste of time. I' m saying, identify the reasons why they are saying these things. They are threatened by your wanting to better yourself. They are self-consciously judging themselves as incapable of making these changes for themselves. When they challenge you with this negativity, offer to have them to come with you, help to encourage them to change their habits. If they decline, they are not ready to make the changes they need to achieve the goals they want. Just because they aren't ready does not mean that you aren't, however. Simply tell them that you are going to achieve your goals and you want them to help in the process but you don't want their negativity around you, because this is very important to you. We must demand better from our support network. A support network that doesn't support us 100% isn't a support network at all.

To be successful in any endeavor we must seek to spend time around people who have succeeded in that endeavor. The daily constant reminder that our goals are achievable is in itself, invaluable. When we spend time at the gym with someone who has lost the weight we are trying to lose, and see them succeed, we are prepared to believe that we can succeed too. This motivation will be the difference between whether you make it to the gym after having a tough day or go to a fast food restaurant. Additionally, developing relationships with people who have already succeeded is a jolt to our ego. If they succeeded, it will be that much harder for us to give up. These people who have already succeeded are the experts. Everything that we are going through, they have already gone through. Take the time to accept this, and accept advice from them if they offer it. They struggled as you struggle. They know the successes and the failures as few other people can. It is folly to think you are the only person going through this struggle, people have struggled with it before, and people have succeeded before you. These people are a literal guide to success, and as I have said before we have to utilize any tool available.

Where to Begin

In this chapter, we will be getting into the process of changing old negative habits, and developing positive new habits. We will address addictions to food as best as we can and we will learn how to stay the course to success. I promise that anyone who is committed to this process can learn the habits necessary to not only lose weight but to succeed in any avenue you wish. If 90% of everything we engage in is habit, and we control whether they are positive or negative habits, there is no limit to how successful we can become.

Before we get started however, it is important for you to contemplate what committing to this process entails. The steps to changing negative habits and creating positive habits aren't that hard. The hard part is in the "practice" of the steps. To be successful, we need to fully commit to the process.

Dedication to the process must be a top priority in your life. The habits are coded into our brains; electric pathways are formed as a "short cut" for performing actions. It is not easy to create new habits, and it does not happen overnight. We need dedicated conscious effort to change these habits over a period of time. These changes can be achieved by anyone, but you have to first dedicate yourself to this commitment.

You cannot be successful in creating these new habits unless you are willing to spend the time each day reviewing your successes and failures, giving yourself the positive reinforcement necessary. You have to be willing to spend the time to identify your habits, both good and bad, and discover how to best change these habits to benefit you. You must be willing to journal about your successes and failures every day, as part of a process to focus on the successes, and to remind yourself of what you need to focus on, to prevent the failures. That means journaling each night and rereading your entry each morning.

There is sacrifice in what we are doing. Your life is going to change. We are changing ourselves to become better people. Our relationships with what we do and, who we involve ourselves will change. This is a hard process, and you must totally commit to it. If you want to change, you will change. I will show you how to change, if you decide to change right now!

I want you to remember throughout this process that we are taking one step at a time. Don't focus on the long term goal. We need to focus on each day, succeeding in each moment of each day. A journey of a thousand miles begins with a step. The only way we will remain dedicated when we get to within 20 or 30% of our goal, and it seems so far away, is to focus only on the short term goals. We will face small setbacks but we are never defeated. As long as we remain consistent, and resolve to improve day by day, we will eventually achieve every goal we have for ourselves.

It is important that we set attainable goals. When I first started this journey with my clients, they had pretty hefty goals. One guy wanted to run a 5k despite being over 300 pounds. A woman who weighed 350 pounds wanted to be under 200 pounds. These are fantastic goals. However, they are not positive short term goals, which are conducive to remaining committed to changing habits. Instead, we focused on running each and every day a little more, and tracking calories each day, trying to keep within a calorie goal. In the long term, these short term goals allow us to achieve our ultimate goal, but in the short term, they allow us to remain on the path to establishing our new habits.

When you can say that you are committed to changing your daily habits, set attainable and applicable goals, and you will succeed. I list some possible goals in the habits section, if you need inspiration. Really consider habits that will help you reach your ultimate goal.

So how do we succeed when we feel like failure? We all know that feeling, when we are faced with going to the gym, or sitting down on the couch. How do we make sure our mind, in a moment of weakness, makes the right choices?

It is important to be aware that our mind is going to resist the changes to the habits we are trying to create. Old habits die hard is a saying but doesn't quite fit. Old habits don't die at all. They are burned into our minds. We can only address them by changing the reward to the trigger. Habits are burned into our brain, literally. Our brains develop neuro pathways directly between the processes of habits, removing the need for conscious decision making. It is going to be a fight to change our habits. However, through addressing negative habits, by addressing the three parts of the habit cycle, we can be successful. We are fighting biology, and this is an uphill battle.

The mind will look for a reason to give up. Do you ever find yourself making the worst of two possible choices consistently? The mind is programmed to take the easy way, it is genetic. This is why we have habits. What are habits, but shortcuts to completing a task?

Any setback, any choice, and excuse can be utilized by the mind in a moment of weakness to make the wrong choice for us. It is important to be aware, that it is at these moments of weakness that our mind will try to justify the wrong choice. We won't always win this battle with our mind. We can do everything in our power to win by preparing ourselves for these setbacks, by limiting choices and by rewarding positive behavior accordingly, but we won't always win.

It is incredibly important for you to understand that minor setbacks are going to happen. You are going to eat too much some days. Other days you won't act in accordance with the habits you want to establish. These setbacks are character building. They are a large part of the success, provided we utilize positive self-reinforcement to identify when and why we made the less than ideal choice and strategize to do better next time.

So, what then are some strategies for dealing with our mind when it wants to give in? The most important thing we can do to combat our mind, in these moments of weakness, is to prepare. Simply by recognizing that these situations occur allows us the opportunity to combat them.

When they happen, hopefully we will recognize these moments of weakness before we act. We should if possible verbally identify this situation. Simply say," this is a moment of weakness", then don't act. Whether you are tired, and don't feel like cooking a healthy meal, or you would rather play a video game than go to the gym. Verbally identify this as a moment of weakness, and then do nothing.

Don't act. Simply refuse to give in to the craving. Identify it specifically, for example if you are too tired to cook so you want to order pizza, don't. Go take a shower, clean something, read a book, do anything, but don't give into the temptation to order pizza. Do this for just a few minutes and you will find that the temptation that was so strong before has is gone. The hardest part is to simply not act on the mind's temptation. Try to accomplish something positive in this moment, something completely unrelated. This provides us with something to acknowledge when we are celebrating our successes. This reinforces positive habits, and the mind's control over us is weaker!

Ok, so you are committed! You want this more than anything and you are going to do what it takes to succeed. Fantastic! But, now what do I do? First thing is first. We need to address any "food addictions" that you may have. I covered earlier in the book food addiction as I see it. I just want to cover some of the bigger points. Food addiction exists, absolutely. In approximately 30% of the cases where I have helped people, in losing weight, there was some type of addiction in the way. The most common was a heavy sugar dependency, usually with caffeine, in the form of soda or sugar laden coffee. Another big issue was with gluten rich foods. That is bread and pasta, as well as cookies, candy and cakes. This is a big one, with the super-morbidly obese, as they often can't control their portions of gluten rich food at meal time. Especially with pasta dishes, while a normal person would be satisfied with one plateful, the morbidly obese person could eat 2 or 3 full plates and eat themselves to sickness. Finally, I have seen chocolate addiction, as well as addiction to salty foods.

Before we can successfully address our negative habits, we need to determine if we may have a "food addiction." This is a necessary first step because we will not be successful in our quest for losing weight until these addictions, if they exist, are addressed. Only you can determine if you may have an addiction, but if you eat a great deal of gluten, or drink a lot of soda, I issue you a challenge to determine whether you have a problem or not.

If you even question whether you may have an addiction with soda or food, I challenge you to give up these food products for three days. Now, the first time I conducted this experiment, I performed it on myself. As I suspected, I had an addiction both to gluten rich foods and soda. It is imperative that you make it the full three days. After that time, I want you to consider your behavior the previous days, the feelings you had. Did you crave more than anything that which you gave up? Did your moods change excessively to the point of it being noticeable by those around you? In my experimentation, I chose to give up gluten to test out my hypothesis that I was a gluten addict. What did I find? The first day was ok, but things started going poorly the second day. Everything was cloudy. I was tired and couldn't focus. I, without even realizing, it started being incredibly short with people because they were annoying me so badly. By the third day, no one wanted to be around me! I literally got into a yelling match with my father, in which I threw a book on the floor, like a child! It wasn't just him. I got into a verbal argument with my boss in a staff meeting. I was short with a couple of my clients I was working with at that point. The fourth day, the cloud had lifted and I was amazed! You don't realize the power something can have over you, until you break the control. It was an amazing experience- being aware that I was so addicted-that this food had so much control over me!

So what was the best part of this experience? Once I broke the addiction everything became easier? Where I once had a hard time monitoring when I ate or how much I ate at a sitting, I was able to control these urges without even trying! No longer did I wait for the next meal or crave more and more of this food, or that food. I would eat a normal sized meal and be full! I wouldn't even start to think about food until I was hungry again. I had broken the control that the food had over me.

So you see if you even suspect it's possible, you need to try to quit for three days. Once you do, you may realize just how much control these foods have over you, and you will decide to make a permanent change. I have all but given up eating gluten permanently. The power over me was too great. That's not to say that when I go out with friends, I won't eat a slice of pizza, or have cake at a birthday party. It is important for you to note however, that with these little trips off your diet, you will have to break the cycle again or you will fall back into the same old habit. It can be hard at times, and I had to develop triggers to remind me of the addiction, so when I did occasionally cheat, I wouldn't give up the changes I had worked so hard for.

The same goes for the other trigger foods. See if you have a problem. See if they have that control over you. If they do, you must make a change. If you don't, you will never be successful in learning these new positive habits, as your mind will never let you focus on establishing new habits when it's craving its addiction. Make this change for yourself. If you can make it three days without the food you are addicted to you, I promise, you will realize just how easy making the other changes can be. Free of the addiction, you will never feel helpless again when establishing new eating habits.

How to Start Identifying Habits

Identifying habits, in itself, is a habit, but it is a fairly easy one to pick up with practice. We must start each day with the intent of learning our habits, before we can make the changes necessary to lose weight, or make any healthy life change. Do whatever you have to, in order to start the day off right. That is, start the day with mindfulness of your habits. Set your cell phone alarm with the title, "Identify Habits". You can sleep with a sticky note on your forehead, if that would work. I actually tried this technique, but I took it off my head while I was asleep Fortunately, for me however, I placed it on my mirror in my bathroom while I was asleep! Whatever it takes, it is important to log these habits if you are to make the changes needed. We must be conscious of identifying habits. Habits are occurring constantly. Our conscious mind isn't consulted before they occur unless we are mindful of what our triggers are, and identify them when they take place.

Do you often get a sudden burst of energy and motivation right as you are about to go to bed for the night? Do you ever suddenly have great ideas or projects go through your mind? The reason we feel so motivated is explained using complicated psychological models. I will explain it like this. It is easy for us to be motivated for something that is a long time away. Have you ever committed to an event that was 6 months away? Or, said in November, you will start going to the gym after New Year's? The same is true for the grand plans we make as we are about to fall asleep. It is easy to promise yourself things, because you aren't required to physically perform these tasks until a later time. The trick is to motivate yourself at that specified time.

It takes effort, in the moment, to perform these ideas in your mind. Often times we will completely forget, as our mind would rather just carry out its programmed habits, and not worry about the changes you considered the night before. We cannot allow our mind the opportunity to push our mindfulness away in favor of autopilot. This is especially a problem when we wake up, as our minds are struggling to wake up fully. Until we are fully awake, our habits take over.

To do this, we must establish habits that require effort by the mind to be conscious of our goal to identify our habits. I am in favor of journaling each night before bed and rereading it again in the morning as the first thing that you do. This will ensure that we are constantly moving forward, each day. I feel journaling is the best way to establish conscious mindfulness when we wake up that we will be working to identify our habits that day. So how do we identify our own habits?

You identify your bad habits by journalizing your activities each day. Do this for a full week. Literally write down everything you do. You can save it on your phone, journalize it online, or simply use a little journal, or piece of paper, such as I do when working with other people. Document when you wake up, what you do when you first wake up. Document when you eat, document when you have your most energy and are feeling motivated. We want to know the good habits and the bad habits that make up who you are.

When you document your eating habits, be specific. Document the time you eat, where you eat, what exactly you eat, whether or not you went back for seconds, who was there. We want to know everything. For example, let's say at work on Mondays, you usually go to a late lunch with your co-worker. You find that when you have lunch with this coworker, you often times will order less healthy food and have dessert, maybe because she likes to eat the less healthy food. Or maybe you do it for another reason? Maybe Monday is an extremely stressful day at your work. It is important to hypothesize the potential reasons because, when we go to change our bad habits, we need to know the cues. Once we know the cues, we can institute better routines to transform our habit.

Transforming Negative Habits

Transforming the negative habits is much more difficult than establishing new habits. However, we can't ignore them. It is the negative habits that have us overweight and unhealthy. This is the failing of diets and exercise programs for weight loss. While they assist in establishing new habits, at least to some degree, they don't address the negative habits that got you to the unhealthy state you are in right now.

If we really want to become a healthy weight, and to live a healthy lifestyle, we need to adjust our negative habits. We don't necessarily have to address them all at once, and some will have a larger impact on our lives than others. It is up to us, once we identify our negative habits, which ones we will choose to focus on. We need to take a good hard look at our habits, and really consider the overall impact changing them will have on our happiness and lifestyle.

If you are having trouble identifying your negative habits, don't worry. We will analyze the most common negative habits that we struggle with, as well as ways to address them. It is very important however, that you independently try to analyze your behaviors and habits, to tailor this plan to your own personal needs. Only you can know for sure what affects you, and how detrimental it is to your long term goals.

So you have analyzed your habits, and have decided which ones are having the most negative impact on your life, with regard to what you want to improve on, whether it is for weight loss, or physical performance, or productivity in school or work. Now we get to work. Remember when we analyzed our habits before; we considered all aspects of the habit. We went over the cues, the routines and how the body is rewarded. To address negative habits, we need to change the routine response to the cue. Really consider what the routine is when faced with a trigger. Now let's consider how to best change this routine to have a positive effect. If the goal is weight loss, the routine is usually food related, right? So in this case, we have several options. The easiest is to replace a "bad" food with a "good" food. We can identify what we eat in that moment, and replace it with an alternative choice, either a healthier choice, or a lower calorie choice. An example would be to replace a bag of chips that consists of 500 calories of oil and salt, and replace it with a small salad with low fat salad dressing, equaling 200 calories. This change, over time would have a large impact on your weight and healthiness. Another alternative would be to replace the eating part of the routine with a distraction, something that refocuses your mind. For example, often, people will eat during a transition in their day. I have had a great deal of success retraining in these situations, by having them refocus on side tasks that will benefit their lives in a positive way. For example, instead of eating when returning from work or school, they would complete chores when they returned home from work, or complete the day's school work when returning home from school, or even reading a book to fill a transitional period.

So, what if we are identifying habits that will help us become a better student or employee? The steps are the same. We identify a negative unproductive routine, such as watching television upon returning home from school. Now, we as students know, that it is best to complete homework when the lessons are still fresh in our mind, so we should complete our homework as soon as possible. We strive to replace television watching during that school to home transition, with completing homework. You will be amazed at how easy the transition is, and how much of an improvement it will have on your success in school.

You may have noticed that the example for weight loss and for becoming a better student is a lot alike. This was intentional. Once you really analyze your habits and realize where you can improve, you start so see areas of your lives that, if addressed, will affect us on several different fronts. It is these "macro" habits that we want to focus on first, as they will have the most positive changes in our lives. As you see in the example, if we change our routine during the transition from work or school to home, we become better students and employees, and we are making healthier eating choices.

So we have identified the habit or habits that we want to change, hopefully with the eye towards having as large an impact as possible. Well, we have identified the habit and how we want to begin to change it. We identified the positives to changing this habit, or how it will benefit our lives, and we have identified the barriers to these habits. Now what do we do?

In striving to make this change, the most important step to success, is establishing mindfulness and accountability to the change. The mind fights these changes and will take advantage of us if we don't remain conscious of our efforts. I am a big proponent of journal keeping, as we began when we started tracking our habits. We must continue writing in our journals each evening. Each evening we will write about the habit we are trying to change. We will be specific about what we are doing, and we will write about our successes, or learning experiences for that day. If you successfully made a better choice of food during your afternoon transition from school to work, celebrate that, verbally if possible. Self-positive reinforcement is a fantastic tool at this moment, as you are very aware of your successes in this moment. Also, write about the struggles you are facing. If you were going to eat a salad for lunch, but a coworker came up and offered you a slice of her pizza and you accepted, write about it and consider how you can address this barrier to success. This will allow you to be better prepared when it occurs again. By writing this information down, it allows you to be ever mindful of the changes you are trying to make and how well you are accomplishing your goals.

In the movie, No Country for Old Men, the main hero in the story discusses the struggle to make a conscious effort to affect positive changes daily. He uses the quote, "We must dedicate ourselves daily anew." We must make this conscious effort for ourselves, to dedicate ourselves daily anew. Too often, do we give up on our well laid plans? Have you ever thought out a diet or exercise plan completely, and completed it for 2 or 3 days and then forgot about it the following day? We have to remain conscious each day about the changes we want to make, as it takes a concerted effort and constant resolve to succeed in changing our habits.

So how can we stay focused, each and every day, towards our goals? This is an incredibly easy problem to solve, as it involves establishing a new positive habit. When I first began really considering the struggle of remaining consistent in the goals of habit change, I realized, why not use our journal as a tool to remain mindful of our goals. So, I started rereading the previous night's entry each morning.

By re-reading our journal entry each morning, we are able to focus on consistently taking steps towards success each day, without delay. This re-reading of the journal, with a fresh mind, helps to keep us focused, and it steels our resolve to succeed. We begin the day focused on something that is very important to us, and we are prepared to face the day with the knowledge that we have the tools to succeed. We have to keep these changes in our consciousness, as it is a great tool in combatting our subconscious' quest to avoid the stress of habit change. Remember, it is in the moments where we lose our focus that we fail.

In addition to our journaling helping us to remain mindful, it is an important tool in tracking our progress daily. This will be important if we struggle with a habit change, as we can more fully analyze why we are struggling with it. If we constantly fail on Wednesday afternoons, when we are spending time with a certain friend or coworker, we will be made aware of it.

Also while tracking our progress, we are consciously aware of how far we have come, and are able to celebrate our successes. We can also identify and learn from our failures. Evening journalizing and morning reading allows us the opportunity, combined with positive self-reinforcement, to maintain the focus we need to succeed in changing these habits.

10 Common Negative Habits

& How to Transform Them

While I feel it is important that each person identifies their own negative habits they would like to change, it is important to explore these habits from a different perspective to get a clear and complete understanding of habits and of the control habits have over us. Even if you went through the process of identifying your habits, I urge you to take some time to read these 10 common negative habits, as it may allow you to consider habits from a different angle.

Negative Speech

Negative speech in the sense that I mean, is that voice in our head we use to approach everything we do, every situation we face, every experience we have. Negativity prevents us from ever really reaching our potential, cutting us off by saying that we are going to fail ,or that we are wasting our time. Negative speech is just our subconscious trying to keep control, to prevent us from engaging in new experiences, where the outcome could cause the subconscious some discomfort. We all do it to ourselves. Whenever there is something we don't want to do, we will be negative about it. For example, there is a person we would rather not spend time with-we speak or think negatively about them to justify our own feelings and actions.

There are many common triggers to that negative voice in us. Our mind uses it as some misguided sense of protection, so anything new may be a trigger. It is different for everyone but you should consider any of these situations. Perhaps undergoing a new project for work causes some form of negativity in you, or performing in school activities. This negative voice defeats us before we even try, in so many aspects. What about that negative voice saying you don't have a chance with this person, or you could never succeed in that as a career? Self-analyze, notice how often, before you even begin, that voice inside your head is determining the outcome.

The outcome of anything is never certain until the finish line. We need to address this negative speech, as it holds us back from greatness in our lives. We can transform this speech however.

Following the steps of addressing any habit, we identify that this is a problem. We become aware of when it occurs, and when we realize the negativity is creeping up on us, make a mental note that we are holding ourselves back. We can utilize verbal positive self-reinforcement in this case, stating that we will have a great experience, or we will learn a great deal. Remind yourself that while you will do your best, the outcome isn't the most important part of an experience.

For one day, concentrate on every word you speak and every thought you have. You may be astonished by how many of your words are negative in nature. Decide you are going to make a conscious effort to replace these negative thoughts with positive ones. Do this out loud if possible. Take care of the obvious ones first. Change every "I can't" to "I will," or at least "I will try." Instead of saying "There is no hope" say "there is an answer, I just have to find it." Change "I can't do anything right" to "I can correct any mistake I make."

Practice this change in habit faithfully and I guarantee you will begin to have a new outlook on life; a new perspective on any difficulty you may face. Suddenly life will become worthwhile, barriers will show a solution, you will have the focus and confidence to take that first step, and then another, and then another. These changes will allow you the personal strength to succeed, whether it be in weight loss or any other aspect of your life that you are struggling with.

You have to be prepared, however, for when there are failures. We have to be conscious not to let any failure we have, or lack of success reinforce the negative voices inside of our head. When we fail, we must identify the positives; what we learned, or how great an experience was. In always taking the positive from any situation, we have the tools to fight back against this voice.

Mindless Eating

Mindless eating is a very common barrier to successfully losing weight. Losing weight is a scientific process. We know that if we eat less calories than we burn, we are going to lose weight. The problem is we don't take the proactive steps needed to track how much we are eating. Whether it be the snacks we eat after work, or a second helping at dinner because we are having good dinner conversation, to the 1 2 3 or 9 drinks we have when we go out with friends, failing to have control over what we eat regularly is THE contributing factor to obesity. If we aren't mindful of what we are eating, we won't successfully lose weight.

There are many times during the course of the day where we often habitually eat without considering the consequences. Some of the most common are revolving around our work day. For example, a lot of us, the first thing we do when we leave our house in the morning is to stop to get a coffee or a soda, maybe a bagel or a doughnut. After all, people say breakfast is the most important meal of the day right? What we aren't considering is that the coffee we got could very well contain over 500 calories, that big gulp soda, 350 calories. Both the bagel and the doughnut are another 300 calories. At break we hit the snack machine for something to munch on while we socialize with our coworkers. Then we go out to lunch with our coworkers to celebrate some goal being completed, or have some cake to celebrate a coworker's birthday. Before we know it, we have consumed 1200 to 1500 calories without even realizing it. This doesn't leave a lot of room for a healthy dinner or any snacks that you eat habitually when you get home.

This is a burden for the obese, because everyone eats habitually. We who are overweight just struggle with eating too much, habitually. We can address mindless eating however. We do this by establishing the habit of planning everything that we eat. We plan the night before, what we are going to eat the following day. At the very least, this plan will keep us mindful of what we are eating the following day, even if we don't stick to our plan completely. Planning what we will eat the following day, along with addressing the habits we listed above, such as replacing the 500 calorie coffee with black coffee, replacing the soda with water, or replacing eating out with a healthy salad, we can successfully prevent ourselves from mindlessly eating hundreds of unnecessary calories each day.

You won't always catch yourself. There will be times, especially when just starting out, when you will eat without thinking about it. Remain consistent. Constantly plan your following day's meals. Strive to stick to only eating what you plan on eating, and focus on making healthy and lower calorie choices. Reread your journal in the morning, refocusing your effort to remain committed to your new eating habits. Eventually, you will establish the habit of being mindful of everything you eat. In being mindful, you will successfully gain the tools necessary to lose weight.

Wasting Time

"If time be of all things the most precious, wasting time must be the greatest prodigality."

~Benjamin Franklin

What we don't realize most often is that our wasting time is a grave negative habit, or habits! If you find yourself wasting time, watching television when you should be doing homework, or wasting time on the internet when you wanted to be exercising, it is because of established habit. The reason you get on the computer and waste a couple hours instead of being productive is because it is your habit to do so. Wasting time is what I called a Macro Habit, that is addressing the habits related to wasting time, will benefit your life in many ways. By identifying, when in the day you waste the most time, then change your routine to be more productive, you will not only benefit yourself in the area you feel is most important, such as being a better student, but you will find that this change of routine will better prepare your mind for the stresses in other parts of your life.

The common triggers for wasting time are anything that can be a distraction, like a cat with a laser pointer; humans are attracted to lights, sounds and actions. We seek entertainment, as it gives us pleasure with very little effort. Remember the pleasure principle, the mind seeks out pleasure and tries to avoid discomfort. To avoid these distractions, identify the common causes in our lives. Computers, cell phones, televisions and music players all have the ability to distract us if we let them. When we are near them, we begin a routine, whether we begin browsing Reddit for two hours, we start playing a Facebook game on our smartphone, or we start watching a reality television show. These routines need to be addressed to affect this change, and prevent wasting time.

The best solution when faced with a distraction, especially the ones we face today, is to just shut them off. Schedule a time when you want to be productive and remove all these distractions. Yes, even remove your phone from your presence.

Distractions happen. In our world today, we are inundated with a barrage of too much information. It is truly information over-load and our minds are in a constant state of stress, trying to absorb as much as possible. To be the most effective person we can be, and to prevent wasting our time, we have to decide what information we want to focus on retaining, and take the steps necessary to do so.

Procrastination

On the surface procrastination and wasting time might look to be the same negative habit but if you go deeper, you will under-stand more fully my meaning. It is important, when striving to live a healthy and successful life, so we must focus on our prior-ities. Often times when trying to lose weight, we will work out for two hours every night for a month straight, to the point of burn out. But in all this time, we never address the food we eat as being a principal cause for our being overweight. We must take the time to prioritize our tasks in life so that we are focusing on what's important. Then we must avoid choosing the easiest task, procrastinating on performing the difficult tasks that lay ahead of us.

Many of us struggle with procrastination; we hear it all the time. What is procrastination but putting off that which is necessary. So how do we address this negative habit? There are different techniques, but first we should identify how we procrastinate. When we have a project due for example, when we find ourselves distracted, what are we doing? This is our routine. The cue is having to work on a project that is going to be due. The routine is to partake in another activity, aside from our project. The reward is performing an activity that causes the mind joy, instead of the drudgery that is focusing on that project.

So we might focus on both the routine and the reward in this case. Let's first eliminate the distractions that allow us to so easily procrastinate. Let's go to a room without television, computers, phones and music. Isolate ourselves with only our project materials. Now we must strive to limit the drudgery of the project. Let's break our project up into sections. Then we can allow ourselves a break after we complete each section. This will give the mind a short term goal to focus on. By limiting the pain side of the pleasure principle, and offering pleasure as a reward for completing part of the project, we will find it much easier to concentrate and get our project done.

This process has been proven to be very successful. By bringing this strategy to bear, as part of a positive habit to eliminate procrastination, we can be much more productive and successful in the things we want to accomplish. We will however, still be unable to focus. We will find ourselves doodling in our book or humming a song or thinking about this person or that activity. If this is the case, and you are unable to focus, simply remove yourself entirely from the situation, leave the project for a while. Not a great time, 15 minutes or a half hour. Do something physically demanding or something tactile to give your mind time to relax. Then proceed to try working on your project again, following the aforementioned strategy for addressing procrastination.

Lack of Personal Accountability

As we strive to make permanent positive changes in our life, we have to consider what habits are keeping us from achieving our goals. There are many and they are varied. One of the most important is the lack of personal accountability. So often, we would rather blame a situation that we are going through, or another person, for a failure in our life. We blame teachers for a poor grade, or our bosses for not receiving a raise or a promotion. We irrationally subconsciously blame family members for us being overweight, as if they somehow contributed to putting the food in our mouths. We blame some circumstance, such as a medical issue, for an inability to be healthier. In this life, one of, if not the greatest negative habit we face is lack of personal accountability. People who succeed are able to avoid finding excuses. They are able to focus on solutions to the negative things we do. As long as we find a way to blame anyone or thing, other than ourselves, for our current situation, we will fail.

We must identify when we are lacking this accountability. When we make the decision to eat cake at work, we have to own that decision, and verbal reinforcement may be necessary. Until we own the choices we make, we cannot succeed in permanent positive changes. We often show a lack of accountability when we are struggling with a goal or a habit change. It is our mind looking for excuses to make it ok to fail. T defeat this habit, we must utilize positive reinforcement. When our mind tries to justify skipping a workout, or ordering a large pizza for our self, we have to be mindful of our mind trying to be weak. Then we can verbally say that if we are going to order this pizza, we are making that choice, and we know that it will set back our weight loss goal. This is often enough to defeat the internal fight with our subconscious craving.

You won't always succeed. You will give in to your cravings and believe your mind's justifications, sometimes. When you realize it, just identify it. Take time to write it in your journal and consider how you can better fight the urge to give in again. Eventually you will begin to consistently win in this struggle.

"Food Addictions"

I want to start by saying that food addictions are real. I have experienced and struggled with them, and I have seen many examples in my work with others. Before we can attempt to counter food addiction, we must first understand food addiction. Food addiction is simply a habit. Unfortunately the cravings are strong, like the cravings a smoker has for a cigarette. The brain needs that chemical fix, which is the reward offered to the brain. This makes it incredibly difficult to fight the "addiction" but we can fight it. To identify this habit, look towards food you consume constantly. Very common ones are soda and grain products, such as cakes and brownies, cereals and pasta's. When you drink a soda, are you able to limit yourself to just one? Can you go a day without it? Can you say the same thing about grain products, or any other food you feel you may have a problem with? "Food addiction" is easy to diagnose. I challenge you; if you feel you have a problem with a food addiction, go three days without the food in question.

The first time I attempted this strategy for addressing my grain addiction, I couldn't believe it. It was to that point in my life, the hardest thing I had ever attempted. Cutting out grains completely changed me as a person. I was moody, arguing with everyone, very emotional and short with people. I was tired all the time and was constantly craving grains of any type. I would salivate watching a pizza commercial, and a couple times I almost gave in and went to the store to buy grains. If I had had any in my house at the time, I would have caved. After three days, the fog that had covered my head lifted, and I was a new person. I suddenly became aware of the level of control this food had had over me for as long as I could remember. It was a sobering thought, that a food product could have that much power over you, as much as any hard drug could.

Once I defeated my addiction, everything became easier. Changing old habits, developing new habits became easier. Once I had broken that connection, life became easier, clearer. I was able to focus on my goals, daily, without distraction. It was the single defining moment on my journey to change. If you think you may have a food addiction, try going for three days without. Notice how strong you will feel after. Do you have to give up the food you are addicted to forever? I occasionally will eat grain products if I go out with friends, or for family celebrations. I still struggle to regain my power afterwards though. Like an addiction to anything, once an addict always an addict. You have to understand to the deepest level, the power that this food addiction holds over you.

Emotional Eating and Responses

Emotional eating is eating for reasons other than hunger. We all do it to some extent but it is a habit that usually begins when we are younger and is reinforced year after year. Unfortunately, we all struggle with emotional eating. It is one of the most common habits, but it tends to only have a lasting impact on those who emotionally eat more, and more often, than others. If you struggle with this, the first thing you need to do is identify why you emotionally eat and what you eat. You can do this as part of your process in identifying habits. You can label the times you feel you are emotionally eating. These will usually stand out because when you eat, you can identify the causes fairly easily. If you are eating around meal times, it is most likely because of hunger. Other times, you eat for social reasons, or because a food you like is available. These other times however, like when you had a stressful day, or had a fight with a family member, or you are falling behind in bills and thinking about it often, these are the emotional eating habits that we are looking to address.

This habit is addressed if you begin planning all of your meals and when you eat. You prevent yourself from eating simply because you didn't plan for the food. You will still receive the craving, so it is important to identify the craving, label it as an emotional issue, and move on using the techniques in this book. Another way to identify with emotional eating is if you feel the NEED to have food right now, as opposed to hunger, where it will continually get worse but you don't NEED the food right at that moment. Once you recognize that cue to eat due to emotional stress, you need to change the routine, of eating that comfort food that you crave. The most effective replacement for eating in this scenario is some form of exercise. You can go for a walk; you can play with your dog. Any exercise you can do will be enough to replace the chemical enjoyment your mind is used to receiving from food. With enough consistency, the exercise will replace the craving for food when you are having an emotionally charged moment. If you successfully apply this strategy to your emotional eating episodes, you will completely change your life, 100%, for the better. You will lose weight, you will handle your emotions better, and you will be far healthier. This is a macro habit to address and I urge you to consider this if you feel it may be a big part of your problem with overeating.

Food Culture

The next common habit we are forced to consider, if we are looking to make positive healthy changes and lose weight is the food culture we currently face. Wining and dining as part of a "healthy" social life is nothing new. In fact, for hundreds of years in cultures all around the world it was not uncommon for people to celebrate with each other over food and drink.

The difference between then and now however, is that we as a culture, at least in the United States, are partaking in this food and drink celebration more often. Also, we are eating an unhealthy amount of calories when we do. Thirty-three percent of United States citizens eat out more than three times a week, over 10% eats out daily. If you add to that the fact that the average fast food meal is over 1200 calories, we have a recipe for the obesity epidemic that we are facing, and a problem that is getting much worse.

Our entire culture has grown to surround itself around food. We eat out with friends and family all the time. Any big event, promotion, birthday, and holiday we celebrate how? By having special meals, or going out to eat or drink.

This makes for an incredibly difficult habit to break, because to address it means that we would have to, at the very least, change how we interact with our social circle, at the most, we may even have to change our social circle some. I can't speak for everyone, but I can speak for myself. When I was at my heaviest, I tended to surround myself with people who had the same negative eating habits as I did. It was comfortable to eat massive amounts of food with other people who would do the same.

So we have to decide how to approach this habit. We can stick with preplanning all meals, even the ones we have when we go out with friends. That's a start, but we also have to prepare how we will handle the surprise invitation. Things are easier now that most restaurants have their menu online. You can search for the healthiest option on the menu from there. So what about alcohol? It is important to know that alcohol can contain a very large number of calories, and depending on your propensity for drink, you may drink up to 30% of your recommended daily calories in a day in one night out.

Communicate with the people closest to you. There is no shame in making healthy choices and positive changes in your life. Tell them you are trying to cut down on eating out so much, or plan when you will go out for a drink. When you do go out, limit the amount you consume.

Apathy

Apathy is a negative habit as well! Do you drudge through life, going day to day without enthusiasm, without focus? This comes as part of our routine lifestyle, a lifestyle lacking any goal or purpose. Apathy is something that we all face at times, but at its worst, it can become habitual and all encompassing.

We need to create in our mind the outcome we want to achieve. Instead of saying, I need to lose weight or get healthier or exercise more. We need to imagine how doing these things will offer us an enjoyable outcome. This is the only way to defeat the feeling of apathy. We need to find purpose in what we are doing. When we are having a sluggish day, we need to consider, is it just a lack of focus on our goals? Being aware that we are being apathetic is fairly easy, as our entire mood betrays us. It's what we do when we are having these feelings that determines if we overcome them to have a successful day, or if we set our goals back by a day.

Obsessing about Others

To end this list, I wanted to touch on one of the most detrimental habits I experience on a regular basis. Whenever I see people struggling with lifestyle choices, whether they are struggling with weight issues, or just healthy habits in general, I come across people who focus on others far too much. They focus on others successes with disdain, they celebrate others failures. They gossip, fight and single out others for their behaviors. This is not the habit of someone who will be successful in changing their habits. When you meet successful people, in career, in athletics, in academics, you can be sure of one thing. They strive to improve themselves, and focus internally, rather than focusing on others. Self-focus is required to achieve the healthy habits that we are striving for.

We have to hold positive internal thoughts to be successful. We do this by focusing on our successes and learning from our failures. These changes require great mindfulness. How can we dedicate ourselves to becoming the best versions of ourselves possible, if we spend more time focusing on others than we do on ourselves? These negative and distracting behaviors keep us from success. So how do we address them?

None of us set out to worry about what other people are doing. It is just easier to judge others for what they are doing than to commit to the effort to create real change for ourselves. We can identify when we are doing this by committing ourselves to self-focus. Part of this is using our journal each night and re-reading it each morning. This allows the self-focus needed for positive change.

When we find ourselves in the act of being focused on someone else and their actions or behaviors, we should identify their behaviors and instead of judging them and obsessing about them, use them as a learning opportunity, of what to do, or what not to do. We need to constantly remind ourselves, to be mindful that we each have our own journey and we need to expend as much energy as possible on improving ourselves, if we are to become successful.

Facing Setbacks

Failure is a part of life; in fact, people fail all the time. Every single person who ever succeeded at anything, failed many, many times before their success. It is this failure that allows us the opportunity to be successful. In fact, without failure, how would we learn what to do versus what not to do?

The secret to approaching failure is first to accept it, and then to understand how productive a tool it can be. Like positive self-reinforcement, and journaling daily, failures play a large part in our progression to the success we seek.

Failure will always lead us in the right direction. After all, with every failure, we can determine how well we are doing, determine problems we will face along the way, and then allow us to plan to face these struggles again. As long as we use our failures to learn from our mistakes, we will always move forward towards success.

So how do we learn from these failures? After accepting them and understanding their importance in the process, we must take the time to analyze them. This is another reason for journalizing the day's events each night. We can look at both our success and our failures. When we look at our failures we, need to consider several factors.

First, is it something that we could have prevented? Sometimes unavoidable things come up. If your goal is to go to the gym at night after returning home, but your daughter had to go to the hospital, because she was sick, this isn't failure, this is something completely unavoidable, and by far more important than missing a single workout. When determining if it was unavoidable though, we must be careful to avoid making excuses for ourselves. We must strive to be absolutely honest, focusing on possible solutions to the failure. Maybe our car wouldn't start when leaving work, so we ran a little late. Did we simply decide not to work out because of a little barrier? We could have probably worked around that.

Next, let's determine how we failed. Did we fail because we were unprepared for a situation? A friend offered to buy you pizza, or you woke up late and missed breakfast? Did we fail because we were lacking mindfulness, and ordered our usual with a coke, instead of the salad and water at our favorite restaurant? Sometimes, we failed because we simply gave in to the temptation. This temptation is almost always the need to emotionally eat. Identify it as you identified the other failures.

Now we can use this information to identify solutions to the failure. Both the friend offering dinner and the missed breakfast are occurrences of being unprepared for potential barriers. A solution to forgetting breakfast might be the healthy fruit you keep on you at all times, or the healthy no sugar added granola bar in your purse. Maybe a solution to your friend offering you dinner is to be upfront before this occurs with your friends about your goals and plans to make healthy changes in your life. What if we failed because we gave in to the temptation? Let's identify that as emotional eating. We gave in to a craving, not the first time it's happened and it won't be the last. So let's look at addressing our emotional eating by identifying the cue, what happened that made us want to cheat ourselves. Then we identify the routine, which was eating something that may not have been the best choice. The best choice in this situation almost always is physical activity. Replace the routine with something unrelated, and reinforce it as a habit you are trying to change.

You see, success can be found in the information you receive after every failure. You just have to have the commitment, the dedication and the desire to analyze them.

Transforming habits is a process. The mind doesn't give up learned habits without a fight and it won't be easy. Remind yourself each night that failure can be a positive thing, and most importantly don't be too hard on yourself when you do fail. As Edison said about failure, "I have not failed. I've just found 10,000 ways that won't work." Be positive about the steps you are making and what you are learning through the process. Remember positive self-reinforcement, it will serve you well.

We all have our good days and our bad days. When I struggle sometimes, I go back to tracking my habits and scheduling positive things in my life to reaffirm positive activity means a positive and successful life. I will usually do it for a week at a time, I have worked with some people who continue to journalize and track daily, even after years. I tracked for a week to refocus myself and I failed to complete my goals on two of the seven days! Now that wasn't ideal for me, but it is important to remember that we are human and we all struggle. The only important thing on this journey is to never give up. If we remain consistent, we constantly strive to better ourselves, we will succeed.

When we make a mistake, when we let ourselves down and fail for completely avoidable reasons it is quite natural for us to get down on ourselves. It is also easy at these moments for us to give up, when we have one bad day we are more likely to have two, two turns into four, and four into ten. We can't focus on the negatives or we will fail. We must, through the process of daily recommitment, strive to make each day a success. If we approach failure in the right light, and strive to succeed each day, eventually we will succeed.

This is going to be a life long journey for us. We must never stop trying to improve our lives and being the best we can be. It won't be pretty! We will face many setbacks as we go and they will come in many forms. We are going to face physical and emotional challenges often. We will face mental and physical fatigue. There will be days when we want to just give up.

What's more, life challenges that we don't expect, sickness for ourselves or our family members, the loss of employment, or struggling with some of the relationships in our lives. We constantly have to fight through these life challenges and distractions. And they come in many forms. They don't always have to be a bad thing. A new child, or personal relationship, or moving for a few career opportunities can be great life experiences for us, but they will provide interruptions in our hard gained changes in habits. We must make doubly sure that we remain focused in these times of turbulence.

Unfortunately, it is impossible to plan for these big setbacks. We can't predict a family illness or an opportunity across the country. So how can we handle these upheavals in our lives while continuing to make positive changes?

We must continuously refocus our minds on what outcome we are seeking. What do we want to accomplish in our lives. Is it weight loss? Or are we seeking success in a career? We must always be cognizant with the end in mind.

We have to visualize the journey. When we plan for the future, we need to look forward to the end goal, but also we have to plan for each step on the way. We have to visualize each step, each barrier and each lesser goal that will add up to the final success. It is important to remember that we accomplish something big through consistent effort.

"A journey of a thousand miles begins with a single step."

Lao-Tzu

We can't get to the end without suffering the journey from the beginning. In fact, the strength we gain from the journey is, in the end, what allows us to succeed. When life gets to be too much, when we face these setbacks, we must take a deep breath and remember, one step at a time, one goal at a time, and one day at a time. If you follow the steps in this book to affect positive changes in your habits, and remain consistent, one day at a time, you will succeed.

To be successful is going to require a certain amount of emotional strength. We are very fortunate however in that the steps we are going to undergo help to build emotional strength! Through our journalizing and refocusing our mind each day on our goals, we will focus on increasing our self-awareness. Self-awareness allows us the opportunity to be aware, not of our activities and goals, but also our emotions. When we understand how our mind is handling our life, emotionally, we are far more capable of carrying on.

With the successful changing of these negative habits, we will gain a positive self-image. As our self-image grows, we will learn to respect ourselves and trust ourselves more. This knowledge that we have been successful, even on a small goal, gives us the strength to strive to succeed in even larger goals. Self-image has the positive benefit of clarity. With it, we will be more able to identify barriers, whether they are food addictions or the other negative habits that are holding us back. This self-image will allow us the opportunity to clearly approach these issues with a clear path to success.

Finally, with the self-discipline that we will build through transforming habits, we will have the strength, the emotional fortitude to face any setback that may come up. The word discipline is really just another word for what we hope to do, establish daily positive habits and perform them consistently to achieve positive results.

Conclusion

We are a product of the decisions we make and the actions we take. All we can control in our lives is how we react to life, the occurrence's that come up, and the goals that we have for ourselves. As I have shown, even those aspects are hard to control, until we have a grasp on the habits that control so much of what we do.

Unless we can control our habits, we will be unable to control whether or not we succeed in reaching our goals. Fortunately, with effort, we can establish a system of positive action that will lead us to a life of success in healthy living. Losing weight will be a byproduct of establishing these healthy decisions.

Changing habits is a complicated issue, and our plans really should be designed for our own personal struggles. If at any time you have trouble identifying your negative habits, or how to address them, I hope you won't hesitate to contact us at our Facebook Fan Page. I will assist you as best as I can, and together we can succeed in making these positive, permanent changes in our lives.